# STILL RISING

# Rising Above the Pain

# Parts I and II

## *"The Experience"*

By


C. BRAYNEN-THOMAS

Printed in the United States of America

First Printing, 2021

Second Printing, 2025

ISBN:

Edited by Todd Larson


Publishing by:

BLACKROCK PUBLISHING BOOKS, LLC
Tucker, GA 30084

The names in this book have been altered for privacy reasons. The accounts described are based on a true story.

Dedicated to my two sons.

# Table of Contents

# PART I

# Chapter 1: Pain was my Normal

At age 11, I started my first menstrual cycle. Every month thereafter, a debilitating recurring cycle of pain would paralyze me for three to four days. The effects of it would often leave me feeling worn out, bloated, uncomfortable, and just plain miserable.

By the time I was 12, I was an expert at recognizing when a cycle was about to hit. I readied myself, canceled plans if I had any, and wallowed in my pain for days. My grandmother and mother would dutifully assist in any way they could, first by making sure I was fully stocked up on heavy-duty overnight pads with wings. (Wings were a must!) My mother would then make me warm soup while my grandmother would get me Tylenol or Midol IB and a heating pad. Usually a long nap or good night's sleep would also help. This worked great when I was safe at home and not so great when I had to go to school.

I attended a small Catholic school in west Atlanta for elementary and junior high school. My family was a stickler on good attendance, so I rarely stayed home from school. In fact, I won perfect attendance awards several times during elementary school. In later years, however, I began to miss more days from school. If "that time of the month" arrived during school hours and the pain was severe enough, I would ask to be excused to the secretary's office (the secretary doubled as the school nurse). Raising my hand, I would get the teacher's attention.

"Yes, Jessica?" she would ask.

"I'm not feeling well," I said. "May I go to see Mrs. Brown?"

"Sure, I hope you feel better soon. Just finish your reading assignment at home. Take care, Hun." And I would be given a hall pass to go to the nurse's office.

In her office Mrs. Brown had a big, fluffy, soft couch on which she allowed students who weren't feeling well to lie down. Let's just say I made many a trip down to Mrs. Brown's office and lay down many a time on that big, comfortable sofa. She was generous with her time and attention, plus she offered me very helpful advice.

"Jessica, I'm so sorry you're not feeling well," she would say. "Lay down and see if you can get some rest. Also make sure not to drink milk while on your cycle. It makes your symptoms worse."

I don't know if the milk theory was accurate, but I really appreciated her attentiveness and love. At her urging, I would lie down on her couch for a while. If I didn't feel any better, she would call my parents to come and pick me up early. Possibly, I would stay home the day after that just so I could be 100 percent well the following day.

Painful periods were the norm for me. They were a part of my everyday life. They were something I accepted and planned for. Furthermore, they came with side effects besides menstrual cramps, including diarrhea and headaches. Little did I know I had been undiagnosed and untreated for a gynecological disorder that was totally foreign to me called endometriosis. It would be more than ten years before I would learn what endometriosis actually was.

# Chapter 2: Diagnosis and Surgery

I looked up at the department name of the Duke University hospital ward and read 'ONCOLOGY' in plain black letters. At the time I didn't even know what the word meant. I was 23 years old. I had been told I would need to have a laparotomy to remove a cyst that was taking up an area in the right side of my lower abdomen. It had likely been growing slowly for months, maybe even years. Over the last couple of months it had started to become more and more uncomfortable. In addition, abdominal exams were becoming borderline painful, and according to the scans the mass had grown too large to melt away on its own. The cyst needed to be removed—and soon.

At pre-op, I walked into the waiting room to meet the doctor who would soon be performing my operation. For some reason I wasn't nervous at all—a little anxious, but not nervous. Thinking back on it now, I'm glad I knew very little about the risks of an "open surgery" or the possibilities that cysts could eventually turn into cancerous masses if not caught early. Instead, what I focused on were: (1) The mass was localized to just one region. (2) From my symptoms, this appeared to be a disease called endometriosis, which was easily treatable. (3) The procedure I was having was a common operation. (4) I would experience great relief after the large cyst in my abdomen was finally removed.

It was a warm, sunny June day the morning I met my surgeon for pre-op. She was an attractive, smartly dressed 40-something medical doctor with a warm smile. She had studied my file and already seemed very knowledgeable about what needed to happen. This certainly put me at ease. Also, I later learned she was an expert in reproductive surgeries with decades-long experience and an impressive track record.

At the end of our discussion she reassuringly said, "You will be fine, Ms. Jessica. I foresee a very smooth operation for you. I've reviewed your charts, and based on my medical perspective everything should go quite well. We will remove all of the mass, which is benign."

I was very grateful for her reassuring comments. I didn't know what 'benign' meant, but it sounded good to me.

Immediately following the surgeon, in walked in her surgical resident intern, who sweetly greeted me hello. "Hi, Jessica!" she squealed in a chipper high-pitched voice. "I'm Wendy!" As she went on to introduce herself and explain that she would be doing my stitches after the surgery was over, I noticed that she was markedly younger and had a bubbly personality with a broad smile, an infectious laugh, and bright knowing eyes. Her energy was delightful! We talked as if we were good girlfriends that had known each other for years. I really, really liked her, not to mention she was very easy to talk to. So I asked her all of the questions I could think of, which she answered patiently. Both positive women helped me go into the process with a positive mind. I was ready.

On the day of the operation, I arrived at Duke University Hospital in Durham, North Carolina. I emptied out my bladder, dressed into the hospital gown and head-cover, removed my contact lenses, and waited to be taken in. My family had come to wish me well and pray for me before I was rolled in. For some reason, seeing them caused me to become emotional, which led to a rush of feelings and me tearing up a bit. Thankfully, the sad feelings didn't last long.

It wasn't long before I could hear the words of the anesthesiologist counting backwards: "Jessica, I am going to have you count backwards for me, starting with the number ten." I responded with "10, 9, 8, 7..." and then I was out like a light. After that, I don't remember anything at all.

The surgery took four hours. It was long and arduous but successful. Apparently, there was a lot to take out! Afterwards, I was told they had removed enough endometriosis to equate to the size of a large grapefruit. It was one enormous chocolate cyst all localized in, on and around my right ovary and appendix. The offending ovary (and my appendix) had to be removed during surgery, since they were visibly damaged. Subsequently, I had to take a couple of hefty shots of Lupron Depot to "flush out and melt away" any remaining displaced endometrial tissue or adhesions. (Let me just add that Lupron Depot had crazy side effects! It made my body feel as if it were in a menopausal state, which caused me to have wild mood swings.) I felt the odd side effects from the Lupron Depot for a total of six months. After they passed, the endocrinologist gave me yet another Lupron

Depot shot, after which the side effects, compared to the first shot, had tapered off somewhat.

After my surgery, according to my doctors, I was as good as new! The surgery and Lupron treatments had been a complete success! Aesthetically I was very pleased at how my scar had healed. Because Wendy had stitched it so perfectly, it had healed into a neat little imperfection. And get this—the scar was shaped in the form of a 'smiley face.' It was oddly quite beautiful.

After the surgery, I was put on Lo/Ovral to manage my estrogen levels, to prevent the growth of further tissue and keep the endometriosis at bay.

The repercussions and long-term side effects of all of this didn't seriously hit me until days, weeks, even years later. For example, the summer after my surgery, I was messaging my good friend Tia about some things that had been on my mind.

Girl, I've been feeling so uneasy.
About what?

> Ever since the surgery and all these birth control pills, I now have to take, I feel a little different. Plus, I've gained weight.
>
> Jess, you're kidding right? You look great!
>
> You haven't seen me lately! If you had, you wouldn't say that. Anyway, what's been bothering me more is the surgery and the fact that I only have one ovary now. I feel somehow less than. Will I ever be able to have children one day? Did they mess something up in there?

Tears welled up in my eyes.

> Jess, don't let this situation get you down. You WILL have children one day. You will be a great mother. Have faith.

Then Tia began to change the subject to something more pleasant. I was grateful for her kind words. Her words of comfort were just what I needed to hear at the moment.

But over the years I continued to have concerns. I wondered in the back of my mind:

*What will I do about children?*

*Can I ever have any?*

*Will I be okay with just one ovary?*

*Every time I hear the word 'endometriosis,' why does the word 'infertility' follow?*

*What about the effects of continuous birth control?*

*Will my cysts come back?*

*How do you 'cure' this thing?*

*Will my dream of eventually marrying and having children ever come true?*

I had so many questions. At appointments I asked my doctors, but their answers were rather vague and hard to understand sometimes. This is when I decided to read about endometriosis. I purchased books, searched the Internet, and looked everywhere I could find to learn as much as I could about the subject.

# Chapter 3: What *is* Endometriosis, Anyway?

Endometriosis was a term that, before my own personal experience, I had never heard of and could barely pronounce! So what *is* endometriosis, anyway?

Pronounced *en-doh-mee-tree-**OH**-sis,* it is a chronic disease in which endometrial tissue, such as the lining of the uterus, grows in or on other parts of the body. It can usually occur in the abdomen, ovaries, fallopian tubes, bladder, or intestines, but it can implant just about anywhere in the body. The tissue responds to the hormones of a woman's cycle and can build up and bleed every month.

Regrettably, there is no way for this rogue tissue to leave the body, which leads to a variety of side effects. Internal bleeding and scarring, formation of adhesions, growths, and cysts (e.g., ovarian cysts), menstrual pains, and interference with bladder or bowel junctions are some of the possible results. Other symptoms of endometriosis include pelvic pain, severe menstrual cramps, fatigue, gastrointestinal upset during menstruation, bloating, heavy or irregular bleeding, pain with or after sex, and headaches.

Endometriosis is also one of the leading causes of infertility and hysterectomy. Regarding infertility, about a third of women with infertility have endometriosis. Among women with endometriosis, about 40 percent are infertile.

Endometriosis can be diagnosed only through laparoscopic surgery, which is exactly what occurred for me. Treatments exist, but there is no definitive cure. My personal experience with endometriosis, in many ways, mimicked the issues many other women experienced.

Moreover, the more I read up on the subject, the more I understood my disease and how to properly manage it. For me, taking certain medications, limiting greasy foods from my diet, and drinking plenty of water helped my symptoms profusely. On the other hand, whenever I did happen to slip and eat poorly, the cramps and menstrual pain in my lower abdomen would become severe and could even sometimes be felt in my knees. Yes, my knees! I can recall many a time when these and other symptoms would paralyze me for days, making me feel just miserable.

Yet I am grateful that, as I became more adept at dealing with the symptoms, the disease itself was not as debilitating. After a while, I knew exactly what I needed to do to manage the pain and live a better life. Once I hit my thirties, I began to shift my focus toward doing what was necessary to preserve my fertility.

# Chapter 4: The Tick and Tock of my Biological Clock

The year was 2014. A year had passed since I had married Thomas. And to date I had still not gotten pregnant. Now I was 37 years old and, according to the medical community, had already reached advanced "geriatric" maternal age. I knew I had better get a move on! The clock was ticking and fast.

In addition to already being on the cusp of advanced maternal age, I had a complex medical history. I had a history of endometriosis, and my gynecologist now suspected a light touch of adenomyosis. As if that weren't bad enough, I had only one ovary as a result of an oophorectomy done almost 14 years prior. The odds were certainly stacked up against me.

So I appealed to my gynecologist, Dr. Asha. A world-renowned Fellow of the American Congress of Obstetricians and Gynecologists, she had studied in Moscow and worked under some of the world's most esteemed endometrial surgeons. Dr. Asha had treated tons of patients with gynecologic issues like mine. Furthermore, her focus was on the study of endometriosis on women. I knew that, if anyone could help me get pregnant, she could!

I remember the day I inquired about getting pregnant. I first informed the nurse who came in to triage me. "I am interested in getting pregnant," I announced. "I've been married for a little over a year. I'm thirty-seven years old, and I'm ready." The nurse nodded intently and scribbled down some notes for the doctor.

When Dr. Asha came in, we discussed my concerns further, including my history of breakthrough, heavy bleeding, and severe menstrual cramps. She said the first thing she wanted to do was to review my previous exams, take specimens from me to test, and do a vaginal ultrasound, which she could do right there in her office. I eagerly obliged. Last, she went over ovulation and how to determine when I have been ovulating. She recommended getting ovulation test strips. Then she advised me to make sure Thomas and I were doing what we needed to do often and at the right time. To top that off, she recommended I lose some weight.

Just as I figured, this wasn't going to be a quick process at all.

Per Dr. Asha's recommendation, I did all she had advised. I counted my calendar days closely, predicting ovulation dates. I went on a diet and increased my exercise routine—the whole nine yards. I was the healthiest I had been in years! Basically, I had done all she had asked me to do. I even went through a hysteroscopy, a procedure that looks inside the uterus using a hysteroscope. When you add together all I had received—the numerous transvaginal ultrasounds, pap smears, abdominal MRI and cat scan, the hysteroscopy, ovulation monitoring, prenatal pills, blood tests, losing weight—I passed every test I took. All "appeared" to be okay.

However, there was still no positive outcome. Still, I could not get pregnant. *What gives?* I asked myself.

The memory of the surgery I had undergone at age 23 rang in my head. *It must be because you only have one ovary left,* I said to myself, and began to worry. I prayed hard for a turnaround.

On my next visit to Dr. Asha's office, this time I met with her nurse practitioner, who told me to try metformin for a duration. It had been proven to improve fertility in women. I was willing to do what it took, so I tried it, and the side effects were horrible! Initially the drug caused me to have extreme diarrhea. Then, after I finally got over that problem, I began to gain weight. I was over it. I officially hated Metformin.

I recalled that Dr. Asha had mentioned a fertility specialist named Dr. Cabernet. I filed the name in the back of my mind. Also, from a certain reality show on TV I had learned about GRS Fertility Specialists in Atlanta. After looking them up online, I realized later that this was the same fertility clinic my gynecologist had recommended. I saw all of it as a "sign" that this was where I needed to be. I eagerly made my first appointment around August 2016.

# Chapter 5: Not Quite Ready

My husband and I anxiously waited in the retro-modern-styled lobby of GRS Fertility Specialists. We were completely oblivious to the fertility treatment process and were excited to learn about it.

Once we were called into his office, Dr. Cabernet greeted us, "Gooood morning, Mr. and Mrs. Vincent!" with a pleasant smile, cracked a joke to break the ice, and proceeded to ask how he could help us. I responded by giving him a long, dramatic rundown of my medical history and mentioning that Thomas and I had been married a little over two years and still nothing. I showed him all my gynecological medical records, told him about my past surgeries and prescribed medications, and more.

Dr. Cabernet nodded as if he knew what I was going to say before I said it. Clearly, this wasn't his first rodeo. He reassured me that, from a fertility specialist perspective, I was still "young" and they got endometriosis sufferers all the time. I was pleased to hear this! My dream of becoming a mother was coming true!

As I heard the many different options, I instantly became excited. Both Thomas and I were ecstatic at the possibilities. This seemed like the best place for us! That is…until we visited the financial counselor.

We were given a ten-page packet inside of a sleek, shiny purple-and-white-colored folder. We skimmed over it as the counselor rattled off a number of different in vitro fertilization (IVF) options and their respective costs, ranging from $5,500 all the way up to $30,000, all private pay.

Thomas and I were dumbfounded, almost brokenhearted. How would we ever pay for this? We locked eyes, gave each other a look, said "Thank you" without signing anything, and proceeded out the front door.

"Hecks, naw! We can't afford that!" I said to my husband once we had gotten into the car.

"Yeah, that was ridiculous," he answered, shaking his head.

Once home, I left the fertility materials we had received in the office in the back seat of my car. There had to be a better way...right?

# Chapter 6: A Second Opinion

I frequently prayed to God about my situation. I asked Him for healing and guidance. I then looked for signs on what path to take. My husband suggested getting a second opinion from another gynecologic specialist. After researching a few online, I happened upon an endometrial specialist named Dr. Jeffries. As it turned out, he happened to be Dr. Asha's mentor, which meant he knew his stuff. I made my first appointment with him.

Despite a positive reception in Dr. Jeffries' office and good vibes from the doctor himself, I initially wasn't overly impressed. He seemed to move even slower than my previous specialist (Dr. Asha). Plus, nothing he had found in the various tests performed had revealed anything new. In sum, I had no new cysts or displaced endometrial growths. My uterus appeared healthy, as did my sole ovary. Overall, Dr. Jeffrey couldn't deduce why I hadn't been successful getting pregnant, nor did he have any "magical fertility treatment or product" I could take. From his perspective, I was in good gynecological shape, all things considered.

The one useful thing Dr. Jeffries did bring to the table that no one else had mentioned was Thomas. He recommended that Thomas, who was seven years my senior, do a sperm-count test to rule out any possible issues on his end. Dr. Jeffries' nurse arranged it to be done at a partnering hospital. I was very grateful to Thomas for taking time off from work to go through with it. He was a complete gem through-out the entire process!

After he had his sperm count success-fully analyzed, we learned that it was in great shape, at approximately 30 million. That said, my husband was definitely not the culprit, not to mention he had an older daughter from a previous relationship who had grown up to be quite healthy. I brain-stormed more ideas on what we could do next.Meanwhile, the fall season had ar-rived. The trees were turning beautiful brown, red and orange colors. The weather was cooler and less humid. It was truly my favorite season of the year. But also, my birthday was in the fall. I would be 38 years old. I prayed even more for a breakthrough.

Acouple of months after my 38<sup>th</sup> birthday, I received a random letter in the mail from GRS Fertility Specialists asking me to return. It came without warning, so I saw it as an unequivocal "sign" to revisit the opportunity of seeing a fertility doctor. *Maybe something could be done to make this thing more affordable,* I said to myself and later to Thomas.

At this appointment we asked Dr. Cabernet upfront if any cheaper alternative treatments were available. He mentioned a procedure called intrauterine insemination (IUI). It was different from IVF in that it placed sperm directly inside of the uterus to facilitate fertilization, whereas IVF involved fertilizing the egg and sperm before transferring directly into the uterus an embryo that has gone through the blastocyst process.

"What are the pros and cons of each?" we asked.

Dr. Cabernet answered thoughtfully, "Well, I will warn you that, for your age range, IUI only has about an eight percent success rate, whereas IVF's success rate is substantially higher. Costs are another variant. IUIs average in the low to mid hundreds of dollars, while IVFs are considerably higher, in the thousands. I know the financial counselor reviewed these with you, correct?"

We nodded, "Yes."

"So it's worth a try to do the IUI, but just keep in mind your outcome is likely going to be better with IVF. I support your decision either way."

Razor-focused on the price tag, we moved forward with the IUI. In preparation, we went through a rigorous battery of tests—and let me just say that the testing was unlike anything I had ever experienced. The clinic tested my egg count, Thomas' sperm count, my AMH, TSH, prolactin, Vitamin D levels, hemoglobin counts, STD screens, immunity to chickenpox, measles, mumps, rubella, Hepatitis A and B, genetic makeup, and everything else you could possibly think of. It was quite thorough!

Then I was put on CoQ10 and Vitamin D, as well as a more highly recommended prenatal vitamin. The testing also found that I needed to renew my rubella shot, so I went to the health department and received a new rubella vaccine.

Once all pre-screening was complete and I had reached a certain date in my menstrual cycle, I went through two IUI cycles. The sweet, patient nurse who was assigned to me walked me through every step of the way. She also ordered and set up each of the prescriptions I would need to take.

On the days of the procedures, everything was quick and easy and lasted all of five minutes each time. All in all, the IUI was not uncomfortable in the least, which relieved me.

We waited the standard two weeks, and then I took my first pregnancy test. Nothing either time.

Chapter 8: Pained

In the March timeframe, Thomas and I began saving up and looking into other ways we could get the remainder of the money together to move forward with a full-scale IVF and FET treatment cycle. We discussed coverage options with our health insurance provider, who at the time didn't cover IVF treatments (but who did begin to cover them after 2017). We discussed getting a loan through our credit union. We discussed grants. We even inquired about military discounts. Last, we discussed redirecting our funds for other bills to this one. It was so very important to me to find a way or make one. And we did. With some creative thinking, we came up with the entire amount through a combination of different sources.

In March, I set up to begin my first IVF treatment cycle and embryo transfer, which included taking additional tests, a prescribed set of medications, and subsequently intramuscular injections nightly for several weeks.

The at-home injection process was where the hilarity began.

I recruited Thomas, who is a licensed nurse, to do the injections for me. The first time we went through this was almost torturous...for us both.

"Okay, Jessica. Stay still, and I will stick you very quickly with the needle," he said.

"Please do it quickly," I responded. "I don't want this to..." Before I could finish the statement, *prick!* I could feel the sting of the needle puncturing my skin. I yelped, then jumped from the sudden unexpected pain.

"Hey, don't jump!" Thomas exclaimed. "See, it's done!"

We both let out sighs of relief. However, both of us could feel our hearts beating through our chests. This process was going to be stressful!

About a month later, the time was drawing near for me to have a pregnancy test in the office. I had completed the treatment cycle, and two weeks had come and gone. I was so ready to see if the process had worked.

Then one Thursday evening, the worst happened. I found red streaks of blood after using the bathroom. I immediately went to the hospital out of an abundance of caution. Later, I would discover that what I had seen that fateful Thursday was the beginning stages of a miscarriage. It was my first time experiencing anything like it.

For several days, the bleeding surged and became heavier and heavier. I went through a record number of sanitary napkins. But that wasn't the worst. The excruciating pain radiated throughout my entire body, and my stomach felt as if it were on fire. I had to take the strongest of pain medicines. At a certain point it got so bad I felt lightheaded and dizzy from the loss of blood. The pain, the bleeding, the headaches were truly debilitating—something I hoped to never have to live through again.

Chapter 9: Starting Anew

After my miscarriage, I went into a brief depression. It was a very sad and difficult time. However, with the help of my faith in God and a supportive husband, I found the strength to rise again. The fight was still left in me, and I was determined to give it another go. I rose above the pain and made a follow-up appointment with GRS to discuss round two, this time with a new fertility doctor in the practice. I am one who always likes to start things afresh with a new experience, new people and new vibes! I was ready for round two!

My new doctor was named Dr. Noble, a female this time. She had a bright, cheery demeanor and bedside manner. I also admired her hip sense of style. She was just an all-around breath of fresh air. She made me feel much more positive as we formally met. "Ms. Vincent!" she said. "I'm glad you decided to try another embryo transfer a second time. We are going to adjust your treatment plan a bit and try things differently this time. And the good news is you have three more frozen embryos."

I nodded trustingly. There was something different about Dr. Noble. Her integrity and positive personality reeled me in at once! I had a good feeling about her "new" approach. I had a good feeling in general.

The first thing I would need was another hysteroscopy, to ensure no "tissue" remained in my uterus from the miscarriage, and to remove any polyps that may have cropped up in the process. Last, the goal was to have a clean slate to start from.

After the hysteroscopy was complete, Dr. Noble and her nurse created a treatment schedule made especially for me. It took into account past and present blood tests and other important markers. Thomas and I followed the protocols to a T, not deviating from them at any point. We had even mastered the progesterone-in-oil applications to perfection. We learned that numbing the skin with ice for several seconds was the key to doing the injections painlessly. The entire process this time around was much smoother, less stressful, and all-around blessed. I was thankful.

Chapter 10: Success!

In June of that year, the best possible answer to my wildest dreams finally came
true. I found out I was pregnant! Not only
did the second embryo transfer work, but
also the embryo thrived and grew and
grew!

I will never forget the way I surprised
Thomas when I found out. Before taking
the official in-office pregnancy test, I
had gone out to a Walgreens near my
job and purchased a test. As soon as I
got home, I took the test and didn't
mention it to anyone. Once I saw the '+'
symbol on the stick magically appear, I
jumped for joy. Still, I wanted to take a
second test to be sure. When I did, I got
the same positive reading. It was time to
share the news with Thomas! I took the
test stick, wrapped it in some decorative
paper, and placed it on the table where
he was sure to see it.

"Hey, honey, what's this?" he asked with a cheeky smile when he saw it.

I just smiled back and said, "Open it."

He did, and as he got to the present inside, his smile turned into a grin. "Seriously? We're pregnant? Jess, that's great!"

We embraced with happiness. The excitement was overwhelming, and I began to feel a type of jubilance I hadn't felt in a long time. I quickly said a prayer of thanks to God, grateful for a second chance.

The next hurdle was getting through the first eight weeks of the pregnancy, after which I could be released from my fertility specialist to an obstetrician. For me, the process of waiting eight weeks was truly nerve-wrecking. This is because prior to this pregnancy, I had only made it to the sixth week. *Would this time be different or the same?* I wondered.

At my two-month appointment, I awaited Dr. Noble's entry into the exam room. Upon her arrival, she and I exchanged familiar looks and greetings, then both of us braced for what we would see on the ultrasound machine. As she held the probe to my stomach, we were both ecstatic to hear the strong beat of the baby's heart. It was the most beautiful sound I had ever heard.

Beaming from ear to ear, Dr. Noble commented, "This baby has a very strong heartbeat!"

I nodded my head, smiling, and said, "Yes! Very strong indeed!"

At the conclusion of the exam, while I was checking out, Dr. Noble stepped out of her office to personally hand me a card with a printout of the tiny image we had just witnessed on the screen. My heart was full, and tears of joy filled my eyes as I read what the card said:

*From the staff at GRS, we want to say CONGRATULATIONS on your pregnancy!*

*       *       *

My dream that had been deferred for years was finally being realized. I was with child. All day that day, and for the remainder of the nine months, Thomas and I were both joyously happy and excited for what was to come. I can remember going to my obstetrician checkups with a surreal, euphoric feeling. It was a feeling I will never forget, and it was one of the happiest times of my life! In those nine months, I collected every single printout I received from the ultrasound tech, vowing to keep them and cherish them for life.

Then, on February 17, 2018, I delivered my first-born love—my miracle-baby, Thomas Jr.! He was delivered by C-section, a healthy, bouncy baby boy. It was truly a beautiful day. And get this: My obstetrician followed the same surgical incision path as my previous surgery at 23—in the shape of a 'smiley face.'

# Chapter 11: I Rose Above

Indeed, the path I took to pregnancy was a road less traveled. It was a bumpy road with many twists and turns, peaks and valleys. It was a pathway full of fear and disappointment, wrought with pain. It was a very long, winding, unpredictable pathway, yet there was light at the end. So I say with one hundred percent assuredness that I would do *all* of it again if I had to.

The experiences in my preteen years to early and middle adulthood did get rough at times. "Period pains" caused me many sleepless nights and depressing days. Endometriosis came with a hefty barrage of new, unfamiliar challenges. Moreover, I experienced a devastatingly painful miscarriage at the age of 38. *Yet, I rose above.* There were many ups and downs throughout my life, and for a time it seemed nothing would ever come easy for me. *Yet, I rose above.*

You see, the dreams I had prayed for did come true; they were just a little deferred. In my case, a dream deferred was never denied; it was only delayed, and finally realized. I am proud to say, with God's help, I rose above the pain and I am finally living my best life, with my loving family.

I continue to rise above the pain!

# PART II

# Chapter 12: Can My Body Handle It?

In 2018, after the birth of my first son, I said to myself, *I would definitely do it all over again if given the chance.* However, as I got older, I began to have doubts. Having a baby, especially while in my 40s, didn't sound as appealing as it once had. Thomas didn't seem to mind one way or the other. But I wasn't as convinced, as I now had friends my age whose children were having children! Indeed, having a child past the age of 40 was not a job for the faint of heart. Could I handle it? More importantly, could my *body* handle it?

Then, in mid-2021, exactly three years after the birth of my first son, Thomas and I spontaneously decided to try for another child. I was 42, and he was several years older. Yet we were determined to give it a shot in spite of the numerical odds set against us! And since nothing had happened naturally in the three years prior—which hadn't surprised me—it was decided that we would go ahead and undergo a third embryo transfer procedure. So far, the odds had been 50-50: (1) The first embryo transfer had resulted in a miscarriage. (2) The second had conduced to the birth of my first son, Thomas Jr.

Praying for a miracle, Thomas and I geared up for a thirdgo.

I reached out to the fertility clinic, and the doctor used the most recent time. Thankfully, Dr. Noble was still working at GRS Fertility, as well as her very efficient team of nurses. They all remembered us from the previous experience and welcomed us back with open arms.

# Chapter 13: Treatment Plan

Thomas and I walked into Dr. Noble's Midtown office one cold Monday in January and voiced our desires about having a child after 40. She nodded approvingly as she patiently listened to my concerns.

"The only concern I have now, Dr. Noble, is not my career, not money, not having a partner to do this with," I said. "It's age. I'm now forty-two years old. Forty-two! I want to be sure I'm still healthy enough and that there are no lingering cysts or fibroids that could block my chances."

"Not to worry, Mrs. Vincent," Dr. Nobel responded. "That would be the first thing I look at. In fact, if you have time, I would like to do an ultrasound of your abdomen right now. That will determine what steps we should take afterwards.

"I just want to add that you shouldn't worry about the age issue. We get so many women your age who go on to have successful pregnancies. The tide has definitely changed over the last five to ten years."

That was the positive response I had hoped for. Thomas returned to the lobby while I went through the examination. It was fairly quick, and afterward we met briefly in her office to discuss next steps.

Doctor Noble notated a couple of small fibroids found during my initial exam, but she said not to worry, as they would likely go away on their own.

In addition, I would need a saline sonogram to assess my situation fully, plus a battery of additional blood tests. That would, then, be followed by an individualized treatment plan just for me.

I was finally on my way. This was going to be a breeze!

Or was it?

"Jessica, you got this." Thomas said encouragingly after our appointment with Dr. Noble. He could sense my confidence level was not high.

"Yeah, I know. *We* got this.", I offered in response, half smiling.

"One hundred percent!", Thomas winked with a wide smile.

*      *      *      *      *

A month had passed, and I had successfully completed the saline sonogram. Following my FET cycle calendar to the letter, I took each of my assigned medicines and shots. Then, within a short number of weeks Dr. Noble successfully performed the frozen embryo transfer. (It seemed as though this time around, the transferal was much easier than the first.) The new treatment plan was well underway. I would continue with the progesterone shots and the daily meds, repeating a similar schedule to the one I'd used before.

Throughout this entire process, I had zero anxiety because, *thankfully*, everything up to this point was so familiar! Not to mention, Thomas was as gracious as always in helping me with the needle sticks, and eventually I got to the point where I could inject the needle in myself.

There was just one problem: the side effects! This time around, the progesterone in oil made me dreadfully sick. Quite literally! Within the first week of taking the progesterone in oil I experienced an unpleasant taste in my mouth, along with an uncomfortable "icky" feeling. It was like a nauseated feeling that just wouldn't go away. In addition, I experienced an aversion to certain foods I had previously loved. My taste buds were literally under attack...and I wasn't even pregnant yet! Indeed, the shots were jolting my hormones into overdrive.

Yes, the side effects were extremely unpleasant, but I decided to press on, with my eyes on the greater prize...a child!

Chapter 14: The News

Several weeks passed. Then, at the appointed time, I went in for the official pregnancy test. The same evening, news finally came in on whether the fertility treatment had worked. Dr. Noble phoned my husband and me with the details.

"Mr. and Mrs. Vincent, hello!" she said pleasantly. "I'm pleased to tell you that you are pregnant! Congratulations!"

"That's awesome, Doc!" Thomas exclaimed. "So awesome!"

"YEAH!", I replied with excitement as my heart skipped a beat. "This is such good news. We really appreciate it." Of course, I had secretly taken a home pregnancy test, so I already knew I was pregnant. But it still felt good to hear the confirmation from Dr. Noble.

That I was able to get pregnant so easily and without as much rigmarole, compared to the first round, caused me to feel a great sense of pride. It brought me sheer joy to know my body was in full alignment and cooperation with the process. The doubt I had felt starting out had finally begun to wane. I was ready for this.

"You got this, Jessica." I said to myself, repeating the words of comfort Thomas had offered me weeks before.

*　　*　　*　　*　　*

Later on in the pregnancy I was brought in for an ultrasound and saw the little tiny baby on a screen for the first time. Everything about it was amazing. Even Thomas was instantly awestruck and excited. "Is it too early to tell what the gender will be?" he asked Dr. Noble as we looked at the sonogram monitor.

"Yes, it is a bit early, Mr. Vincent," Dr. Noble said. At the nineteenth week or so, you will be able to tell. Right now, we are only at five and a half weeks."

"I hope it's another boy."

I cleared my throat. "We will be happy with whatever the gender is," I said sharply, looking over at Thomas.

"Oh, yes, of course." Thomas sheepishly smiled at Dr. Noble and me.

We all laughed heartily.

# Chapter 15: Surreal

The Collins dictionary definition of 'surreal' or the act of having a surreal experience is when elements combine in an unbelievable way that you would not normally expect, much like in a dream. Going through such a surreal experience like this one made me feel like I was literally gliding through a fantasy world in an out-of-body experience. I continued to feel this way over the entire course of this unbelievable journey.

I first felt it when we viewed an image of the blastocyst embryo on the day of transfer, then afterward when we received the call that I was pregnant, as well as when we saw the budding embryo take shape on the ultrasound machine. Many more surreal moments followed. Indeed, this entire experience had been so beautiful, utterly amazing—just perfect! I found myself adoring the small baby growing in my womb, sight unseen. I was already in love.

Indeed, the dream I had been living in had been wonderful leading up through this point. Everything about my pregnancy experience had been perfect, in fact.

But would that continue?

# Chapter 16: A Badge of Honor

$$A$$s the pregnancy progressed, I experienced nearly every possible symptom. To this day I don't know if they resulted from my advanced maternal age (42) or were simply side effects of my endometriosis. Nevertheless, I pressed on, resolute to rise above the pain and discomfort. Trust me, it was quite a laundry list! I experienced:

- Morning sickness
- Food aversions
- Severe heartburn
- Hemorrhoids
- Lightening pains
- Constipation
- Fatigue
- Low iron
- Elevated heartrate
- Subchorionic hemor-
  rhages

I often refer to this experience as my badge of honor because it truly tested my resilience and strength. For nine long months, I endured an incredibly challenging set of side effects that seemed to come one after another. It was nothing like my first pregnancy, which had been smooth and almost effortless—a complete breeze in comparison. This time, however, I found myself second-guessing my decision and seriously wondering whether I had gotten in over my head. Despite consulting doctors, specialists, and midwives, no one could give me a definitive answer as to why this pregnancy was so tough. Still, they worked diligently to help me manage the symptoms, and among them, the midwives stood out for offering the most practical and comforting suggestions.

Here is how I coped with each challenge:

- **Morning Sickness:**
  To combat relentless morning sickness, I made hydration a top priority. Every single day, I drank at least six cups of water to keep my body balanced and reduce nausea. Additionally, I learned about a medication called Unisom, which is often recommended for severe morning sickness and food aversions. Incorporating this into my routine provided much-needed relief and allowed me to regain some sense of normalcy during those difficult early months.

- **Heartburn:**
  Heartburn became one of

my most persistent and uncomfortable symptoms. After trying several remedies, I discovered that Pepcid AC was the ultimate lifesaver. It worked quickly and effectively, completely eliminating the burning sensation that had made eating and even resting a challenge. This simple solution brought immense comfort and allowed me to enjoy meals without constant discomfort.

- **Hemorrhoids:**
  Hemorrhoids were another unpleasant side effect that required lifestyle adjustments. To alleviate the pressure, I spent more time lying on my side and avoided sitting in chairs for extended periods. These

changes, though small, made a noticeable difference. Over time, the condition resolved on its own, proving that patience and consistent care can go a long way.

- **Lightning Pain:**
  The sharp, sudden pains—often referred to as lightning pains—were particularly alarming. To manage these, I invested in a supportive pregnancy belt. This accessory turned out to be incredibly helpful, not only for easing lightning pains but also for reducing general discomfort caused by the added weight and pressure of pregnancy. It quickly became one of my most trusted tools.

- **Constipation:**
  Constipation was another recurring issue, but I found that maintaining a steady intake of water each day usually kept it under control. On rare occasions when hydration alone wasn't enough, I resorted to a stool softener, which provided gentle relief without causing additional complications.


- **Iron Deficiency:**
  Midway through my pregnancy, a blood test revealed that I was suffering from iron deficiency, which explained the overwhelming fatigue I had been experiencing. To address this, I began taking iron supplements

as recommended by my healthcare provider. Once my iron levels returned to normal, I noticed a significant improvement in my energy and overall well-being.

- **Rest and Stress Management:**
Finally, one of the most important steps I took was prioritizing rest and eliminating unnecessary stress. I made the decision to take maternity leave two weeks earlier than planned, giving myself time to recover and focus on my health. This period of rest proved invaluable, helping me manage lingering symptoms and even aiding in the healing of a subchorionic hemorrhage—a complication that had

added to my worries earlier in the pregnancy.

*Note: The above should not be treated as medical advice. All treatments should be approved and monitored by the close oversight of an obstetrician, physician or midwife.*

*      *      *      *      *

Of all the challenges I faced during those nine months, nothing compared to the moment I learned I'd had a subchorionic hemorrhage. The words alone sounded ominous. Medical experts aren't certain about the root cause, but most researchers agree it results from a partial detachment of the outer fetal membrane from the uterine wall. It can potentially result in vaginal bleeding (which is what happened to me), mild pelvic cramping, or no symptoms at all. In my case, I didn't experience

cramping, but I experienced significant bleeding for about 4-5 days.

I remember uncomfortably sitting
in the examination room, clutching
the edge of the exam table, waiting
for answers. The ultrasound con-
firmed the location of the hemorrhage and, to my relief, that the baby
was okay. My doctor explained that
while many subchorionic hemor-
rhages resolve on their own, they can
increase the risk of miscarriage, pre-
term labor, and other complications.
After hearing this, I committed to following every recommendation: bed
rest, hydration, and eliminating
stress. I cleared my calendar, stepped
away from work earlier than planned,
and gave myself permission to slow
down.

Week after week, I watched that
hematoma shrink on the ultrasound
screen. Slowly, steadily, healing

came. And with it, hope bloomed again. The baby continued to grow—stronger, bigger, thriving with every day that passed.

*    *    *    *    *

I rose above the pain and eventually delivered my second baby boy successfully and right on time the following February, at the seasoned age of 43. This, with the help of my obstetrician, midwives, maternal fetal specialists, nurses, Thomas, and God, a baby was born. And in spite of it all, I again said, despite all of the many difficulties I had faced, I would absolutely go through them again.

# Chapter 17: Pivotal moments

The day had finally come to have
the baby. Because of my "compli-
cated" history, it was decided that a C-
section was the right way to go.

So, on that chilly February morning, I changed into my hospital gown
and was wheeled into the operating
room. The sterile brightness of the
lights contrasted with the warmth of
anticipation in my heart. The anesthesiologist greeted me with calm re-
assurance as he prepared the spinal
anesthesia—a medicine designed to
numb me from the waist down. Even
that process carried its own set of
sensations and side effects. Once the
injection was complete, I was posi-
tioned carefully, and soon after,
Thomas walked in to join me. His
presence never felt better and I was
grateful.

When Dr. Penguin and her surgical
assistant began, I felt only the

faintest tugging here and there—a surreal awareness that something monumental was happening. To my immense relief, there was no pain, only quiet concentration filling the room. Occasionally, the doctor's voice broke the silence with words of encouragement: "You're doing great, Jessica! Not much longer now!" Those words were like lifelines, as I waited in nervous anticipation.

And then, it happened—the pivotal moment that would forever be etched in my memory. A loud, piercing cry filled the room, a sound so pure and beautiful it seemed to silence every fear I had carried for nine long months. I had never heard anything so lovely—not since the birth of my first child. In that instant, time stood still. A flood of emotions swept over me—relief, joy, gratitude, and an overwhelming sense of *love*. The nurse gently handed the baby to

Thomas and me, her voice bright with celebration: "Congratulations, Mom and Dad! You have a healthy baby boy!"

Tears blurred my vision as I whispered, "I love him already! Hi, my little guy!" My heart felt like it could burst from the sheer magnitude of love and awe that I was feeling. Thomas, too, was overcome, his eyes fixed on his son with tenderness. "Welcome to the world, my son," he whispered softly, a promise wrapped in love.

We named him Tucker.

*   *   *   *   *

That moment was more than the arrival of a child; it was the culmination of a journey marked by resilience, faith, and unwavering hope.

Every hardship, every tear, every sleepless night had led to this miracle. Tucker's cry was not just the sound of life—it was the anthem of victory over fear, uncertainty, and pain. It reminded me that even in the darkest valleys, light can break through. That love, aligned with faith in God, can carry us through storms we never imagined we could survive.

As I held Tucker close, I realized something profound: motherhood is not defined by perfection or ease. It is defined by endurance, by the quiet strength that rises when everything feels impossible. It is the courage to keep going, even when the path is steep and the outcome unclear. And in that operating room, with my son in my arms, I knew—I had done it. We had done it.

If you are reading this and walking through your own season of

uncertainty, let this be your re-
minder: **you are stronger than you
think.** The road may be hard, but it
leads to beauty beyond measure.
Hold on. Keep believing. Because one
day, God-willing, you too will hear
that cry—the sound that makes every
struggle worth it.

Chapter 18: Musings

The swerving, topsy-turvy journey I took to motherhood was not ideal. I entered the journey with a late start. Not only that, but I didn't even have all of my "members" in place. In other words, I was short an ovary, and, because of the endometriosis that plagued me since the age of 11, I had been diagnosed as medically infertile by 25.

Nevertheless, I persevered! With the help of my spiritual foundation and my wonderful husband, I pressed on through until I rose above the pain. I had not only reached my goal, but I had surpassed it, with two beautiful children to show for it. Our family of three was now a family of four. We, the Vincent family—including Thomas, Jessica, Thomas Jr., and Tucker—were now complete.

Thank you for your support!

THE END

# References


Ballweg, Mary Lou. *The Endometriosis Sourcebook*. New York: McGraw-Hill Education, 2003.

Collins Dictionary. "Surreal experience.", Last edited 2022. Retrieved from https://www.collinsdictionary.com/us/dictionary/english/surreal-experience

Wikipedia. "Endometriosis." Last edited on June 6, 2020. Retrieved from https://en.wikipedia.org/wiki/Endometriosis

<u>www.authorandmompreneur.com</u>

THANK YOU FOR YOUR
SUPPORT!

www.ingramcontent.com/pod-product-compliance
Lightning Source LLC
Chambersburg PA
CBHW072242260726
48657CB00001BA/422